Back to Basics

A short guide to the fundamentals of healthy living

Sid Riley

Table of Contents

<u>Foreword:</u>

My interest in the link between calorie consumption, exercise, and weight began Mid-2016 when I Joined the UK armed forces at 19 years old. I started my basic training weighing in at an average 73KG and at the time considered myself fit and healthy considering I played rugby, training on Thursdays and a match most Sundays.

It was only after the first PT (physical training) session I realised how wrong I was. It was a beasting. A common term in the armed forces but for those of you who do not know what a beasting is, imagine an incredibly demanding and physically intense training session, then multiply that intensity by ten and add a dash of angry, screaming physical training instructors to complete the recipe for what are some of the most arduous training sessions you can do.

By the end of the session, I was more sweat than man and I felt like my legs were going to give up supporting my weight at any moment. The only person who was not gasping for air like a fish out of water was being sick. This really set the tone for what was to come.

I went from having the standard three meals a day to an average of five. Breakfast, snack, lunch, dinner, and another late snack became my daily routine for eating. At the time I thought I probably would not gain any weight as I was eating more but also exercising more. Two and a half months later I completed my basic training and to my surprise, I weighed in at roughly 81KG.

This got me thinking, why?

I am eating more, and my weight has increased but I am also doing a lot more exercise, I am able to run further and lift more than I have ever been able to before. So, what is the fundamental link between food, exercise, lifestyle, and weight?

I have written this book to share my knowledge of why, to help you avoid those plans that only seek to lighten your wallet and provide you a solid foundation of knowledge on which to start your weight loss journey, to change your perception of calories and ultimately improve your overall health.

Chapter 1:

Introduction

The diet and weight loss industry in the UK is worth an estimated £2 billion every year. A drop in the ocean when compared to the United States which is estimated to top $70 billion per year[1]. This incredible amount of money clearly shows how desperate millions of people are to find pill, plan, secret tip, specialty diet, or celebrity fitness regimen that will finally let them lose those unwanted pounds. An estimated three quarters of people in this country are overweight or obese, and many other countries are close behind. Far too many people with weight problems look in all the wrong places or to the wrong people for a solution[2].

The "secret" to dieting and weight loss has been right in front of you all this time. If you eat and drink fewer calories than you burn, you will lose weight. This simple scientific fact holds true for every healthy person, man or woman, old or young.

The Diet Disillusion

The definition of disillusion is "disappointment resulting from the discovery that something is not as good as one believed it to be."

This is an important sentiment as, from personal experience I know it is one I have experienced, as many others will have too. When it comes to trying to lose weight with the latest "fad" diet plans, the results they are said to produce are often unattainable for the average dieter.

Consequently, when those results do not present themselves as quickly as you were told or expected, it is all too easy to become disillusioned with trying to lose weight.

You may think that you cannot lose weight and that is just who you are but that could not be further from the truth. You are not alone in thinking this; each year the average dieter will have 4 attempts at losing weight. And this is the first mistake most make when starting their weight loss journey. Many consider weight loss just a 12-week plan that you follow and that is it.

Losing weight is far more than a set plan over a specific timeframe. It is a lifestyle change and requires a whole new way of looking at food consumption, daily habits, and exercise. It was only when I made my weight loss goal a lifestyle change rather than a few weeks of strict control on what I was consuming that I began to see consistent results.

What is the key to consistent weight loss and control then? It is calorie counting.

The Key to Weight Loss

Calorie counting is the only solution to losing unwanted pounds and keeping them off for the rest of your life.

Every fad diet, questionable supplement, and latest fitness craze is about calorie consumption at their core. They are just cleverly marketed to make your wallet lighter while promising near-magical results in an unachievable time frame. Weight loss is not a 30-day challenge or even a six-month goal. All it takes is a quick search of the internet and you will find article after article displaying varied numbers on how many failed diet attempts there are each year. Regardless of the precise numbers, it is clear that those looking to lose weight fail to understand that a short-term fad diet or pill is not the answer. A permanent lifestyle change and a new relationship with calories is required.

After months or years of trying to lose weight, you may balk at the idea that simply counting calories will get you the results you want. First, it is important to understand what calories are and why paying attention to how many you take in and how many you use every day makes sense. Second, you need to know how to create the right calorie-controlled way of life for you.

Get ready to go back to basics when it comes to dieting and weight loss. You can find the success you want and a new, slimmer, healthier you without wasting any more time or money.

Chapter 2: Fundamentals of Calorie Counting

Calories are not a type of nutrient and they are not intrinsically bad like some people think. A calorie is simply a unit of measurement for energy that comes from foods and beverages.

Scientifically speaking, a calorie equals the amount of energy needed to raise the temperature of a kilogram of water one-degree Celsius[1]. This unit of measurement is used in other types of science beyond nutrition. Unless you intend to work in a lab, you do not need to know the rich history of the scientific process, as interesting as it is.

Viewing calories as a unit of energy becomes easier when you understand that food is fuel. The calories and wide range of nutrients available to consume give your body what it needs to carry out every function from the tiniest cellular repair to large-scale activities from going on a run to gardening and even just sitting around and doing nothing. After all, involuntary processes like respiration, circulation, and digestion need energy too.

<u>Why Calorie Counting Matters</u>

All food and drinks other than pure water have calories in them. Your body needs a certain number of calories to function healthily. To maintain an appropriate weight, you cannot take in more than this amount. Everybody is different and has different calorific needs. Determining your proper daily calorie intake is the first step to make calorie counting work.

A lot of claims exist and state that calorie counting is bad, it does not matter, or it is even dangerous in some way. Comments like these usually show up when someone is trying to sell a new fad diet or fitness programme. If any of them work, however, it is due to a calorific deficit. In fact, research shows that programmes that include calorie tracking result in more weight loss than those that do not[2]. You can skip the expense and complexity and simply count calories on your own.

Calories in, calories out. This simple equation is all you need to know to lose unwanted pounds, reach and maintain a healthy weight, and feel your best now and in the future. It is a simple solution to a serious problem that affects millions of people all around the world.

The Basics of Calorie Counting

Your body needs a certain number of calories to function at its most basic level. These units of energy make it possible for your heart to beat, your lungs to breathe, your digestive tract to process nutrients, and your brain to think and make decisions for you. This is your basal metabolic rate (BMR)[3].

You also need extra calories to fuel physical activity which burns more calories than your body does at rest. If you ask an endurance athlete or bodybuilder how many calories they eat, you may be shocked to hear the high numbers. They need more calories because they are incredibly active. Even if the only physical activity you do includes walking your dog or washing dishes you still need calories to fuel it.

If you eat exactly the number of calories you need to fuel your body, you will not lose or gain weight. If you eat too many, your body stores the extra energy as fat. If you eat fewer than you need, those fat stores are broken down and used as energy again. This is how weight loss works at its most basic level.

Calorie counting needs to become your first new habit for your weight loss journey.

How to Count Calories

The only way to make sure you eat fewer calories than you need is to count them. Many different helpful calorie-counting tools exist, and the one you choose depends on your preference. For best results and to increase the chances of you sticking with your new habit, pick the simplest and most convenient method.

Check Food Labels and Keep a Record

In the United Kingdom, all foods require a nutritional label that includes the calorie count per serving. Although some concerns exist about the accuracy, labels provide sufficient data to keep track of calorie intake if you know how to read them. There are three things to take into account.

1 – Margin of Error – Local Authority Co-ordinators of Regulatory Services (LACORS), the body that advises trading standards officers about enforcing food laws allows a certain margin of error[4]. Nowadays calorimeters are more advanced and accurate however, imprecise calorie counts still happen and are allowed because it is impossible to weigh the exact nutritional makeup of each individual piece of packaged food. Processed food manufacturing companies have a financial interest in making their calorie counts seem as low as possible and may use this margin of error in their favour.

2 – Unrealistic Portion Sizes – Advertising that a snack food has just 100 calories per serving is a great way for companies to attract attention. It looks like an affordable snack in terms of calorific value, but when you look closer at the label, you see that the portion size is unrealistically small. Does anyone really only drink half a bottle of fizzy drink or eat half a packet of crisps the way their portion sizes suggest? Learn more about appropriate portion sizes in Chapter 3.

3 – Natural Discrepancies in Food – One almond is larger and may have a higher fat percentage than another in the same bag. A glass of juice may have a higher pulp or sugar content than the next one you pour. There is no way for the average person to measure these discrepancies without access to a full scientific lab in your kitchen.

Although these issues affect the accuracy of food labels, you need to track something to maintain a calorific deficit. The numbers provided on food labels are more than adequate and accurate enough for calorie counting. Also, if you want to lose weight, eating a larger almond one day or drinking juice with more pulp is not going to affect your diet in drastic ways.

Some people keep a record in a notebook or journal, while others use a spreadsheet or chart on their computer. While these methods work, you might find a phone app or online tracking platform more convenient, especially when you are on the go.

Use a Calorie Tracker App

What could be simpler than taking out your phone at every meal and snack time, typing in your food list, and having an automatic calorie and nutrient record? Multiple diet-tracking apps and platforms exist on the market today, most have a free option too. They usually use a database or other trusted sources for a wide variety of natural and prepared foods and meals. They offer an easy and convenient way to keep track of your calorie intake over time.

Many apps offer water tracking too, so you can keep an eye on how much water you are drinking each day. I will talk more about water and the link it has with weight loss later in this book.

When it comes to calorie counting, the method you use is less important than creating a regular habit, measuring your food accurately, and recording absolutely everything you eat or drink every day. Accuracy and consistency will determine your success in your weight loss efforts.

With the apps available on your phone nowadays there are no excuses for not counting your calories.

<u>Calories Out</u>

Losing weight is an equation. Calories in minus calories out. Making sure you are in a deficit will ensure you lose weight. We have talked about counting calories in but what about calories out?

Generally, calorie consumption is recommended to be 2500 for men and 2000 for women. Although, this will vary depending on your activity levels.

As with counting calories in, using an online or mobile app is the most convenient and effective way to calculate calories out each day. This is made even easier if you have a smartwatch or fitness tracker.

Although it may not be 100% accurate it will be more than suitable for the average dieter.

Chapter 3: Portion Sizes

Increasing portion sizes are one reason for the current obesity epidemic. In countries that traditionally serve smaller amounts, obesity levels are much lower. For example, look at a comparison between fast food portion sizes or large fizzy drink sizes in the UK and the USA. In the UK, a large soft drink is 500ml (17.5 oz) whereas, in the USA a large soft drink is 850ml (30 oz). This is a 70% larger serving size.

When restaurants serve larger portions, calorie intake rises. It also echoes in homemade meals because people get used to eating more. A larger portion size becomes the norm.

When you understand how many calories you burn and adjust your eating habits to stay under your allowed calorie amount, you will find your portion sizes getting smaller. Controlling portion sizes by measuring and weighing ingredients helps you stay in control of your calorie intake. Over time your portion sizes will stop seeming small and will become your new norm.

<u>As Average Portion Size Grows, So Do We</u>

Both accepted portion sizes and the amount people eat has grown considerably over the past decades. It is no surprise that the numbers of overweight and obese adults and children have also skyrocketed. The more food you eat, the more calories you consume, the more excess energy gets stored as fat. It is a logical progression that everyone should understand.

People today eat approximately 200 to 500 more calories per day than they did in the 1970s[1]. Portion sizes have expanded no matter what type of food you choose. Sit down restaurants serve large portions, sometimes sufficient for two people. Fast food restaurants offer super-sized options at highly affordable prices. Packaged snack foods offer more size options than ever before, and even supposedly healthy choices push larger portions.

Clever marketing and insidious portion size creep contribute to societal weight issues. However, it is ultimately up to you to determine healthy portions with appropriate calorie levels. In order to succeed with calorie counting and losing unwanted fat, you must retrain your brain to recognize and feel satisfied with smaller amounts of food.

Examples of Portion Size Growth

Studies conducted about portion sizes over time have shown an overall increase in the average portion size. The main culprit seems to be marketing. When people get more food for their money, they think it is a great deal. Instead of a smaller, healthier portion, they are willing to pay a bit more with promises of increased value.

A late 20th century study by the University of North Carolina quantified across the board increases in portion sizes. For example, the size of a takeaway burger had grown 23% since 1977, all sizes of soft drinks had grown more than 50% and snack food bags increased by 60%[2]. Other studies show similar results. A bottle of beer in the 1970s averaged six ounces while you can easily find 40-ounce options today[3].

These changes were gradual and therefore unnoticed by most people. When offered more food in a package or on a plate, people ate it without feeling any more or less satisfied than they did before. In a way, clever advertising and more product options have brainwashed people into expecting more food and feeling dissatisfied with smaller portions even if they provide sufficient calories and physical satiation.

Choose the Proper Portion Size for You

It would be incredibly simple to have one set healthy portion size that suits everyone. However, everyone's calorific needs are different. First, understand the criteria that go into portion choice, and second, learn how to measure and control how much you eat and drink.

Factors to Determine How Much You Can Eat

A 60Kg woman with a desk job needs a vastly different daily calorie intake to a 95Kg man who works in construction. Many factors go into figuring out calorie levels and portion sizes. Of course, the size of the portions you eat depends on how many calories they contain. When you measure out 75 grams of pasta for dinner, the measurement is much less important than the fact that you are consuming approximately 95 calories.

The five factors listed below help you figure out the right number of calories to eat, which informs your portion sizes for the foods you include in your diet.

1 – Your Current Weight and Size – Taller and heavier people can eat more calories and maintain their body size than short and slim people can. This makes it easier for obese people to lose weight at the beginning as they can still consume quite a lot of calories and still lose weight.

2 – Age and Sex – Men, on average, can eat more calories than women even if they share the same measurements because they generally have more muscle mass and lower body fat percentages. A shift from muscle to fat also reduces the total amount of calories needed as you get older.

3 – Basal Metabolic Rate (BMR) – Maintaining vital functions like breathing and digesting food requires calories. BMR differs for many reasons including body size, age, sex, overall health, and genetic factors. People have different metabolisms, so they need different amounts of calories to live.

4 – Physical Activity Levels – Any type of activity or exercise burns calories. People who do more than sit around can eat larger portion sizes and still lose weight. Of course, a calorie deficit must still exist.

5 – Desired Weight Loss – Since you know you need to take in fewer calories than you use in order to drop unwanted pounds, your portion sizes should reflect this. It may seem that the smaller your portions, the more weight you lose. However, you should never reduce intake to unhealthy levels. After all, you still need to satisfy your BMR and keep all your body systems functioning optimally.

You can figure out your perfect portion sizes and healthy calorie intake with one of many online BMR and TDEE calculators. TDEE stands for Total Daily Energy Expenditure, which represents your BMR plus an extra calorie allowance based on physical activity levels. A general rule of thumb is that no one should eat fewer than 1200 calories to maintain life. Most people can eat quite a bit higher than that and still lose weight. Discuss your specific needs with your doctor, a certified nutritionist, or another expert.

How to Measure Portion Size Accurately

If you want to track calories accurately, you need to measure your portion sizes. Far too many people underestimate how much they eat. In the beginning, use a set of scales and measuring cups to get specific portion sizes. If you eat out at a restaurant, a friend's house, or simply do not have the ability to use these tools, there are some tricks to determine healthy portions.

1 - Food Scales - The best way to measure your portion sizes and get accurate calorie counts is to use a set of scales for everything you put in your mouth. Weigh servings of prepared food and compare them to the amount listed on the label. Measure ingredients when you make yourself a sandwich, cook a full dinner or grab a simple snack.

2 - Measuring Cups and Spoons - Tracking volume is the second-best way to measure portion sizes. This gives you slightly less accurate data because foods fill a measuring cup or spoon differently depending on their size. A cup of dry pasta, for example, may have a different amount of food in it due to the spaces between the pieces. A cup of orzo will have a lot more food and calories in it than a cup of rigatoni.

3 - Size Comparisons - If you find yourself without measuring tools, learn to judge correct portion sizes by eye[4]. A healthy serving of pasta is about two handfuls worth, a baked potato the size of your fist, or a piece of grilled chicken about half the size of your hand. This is an important skill to learn as there will often be times when you are out and do not have any way to accurately measure what you are consuming.

Chapter 4: Cheat Days

I have included cheat days in this book as they are a real bugbear of mine. This chapter will be short and sweet as there is not too much to talk about when it comes to cheat days but, I did want to include them as I find they are something people often fall foul of when it comes to losing weight.

What is a cheat day?

A cheat day is when someone takes a break from their diet plan for a day. The idea is that the dieter can 'cheat' on their diet plan for one day if they stick to it for the rest of the week. Many include a scheduled cheat day each week in their diet plan in hopes of reducing cravings and preventing binges.

What is the main issue with a cheat day?

Cheat days are meant to prevent binging during the week. What happens is when someone on a strict diet plan reaches their scheduled 'cheat day', they cram an entire week's worth of binging, be it food or drink, into one day because "it is a cheat day". This is circumventing the intended purpose of a cheat day. Initially used to prevent binging it is now enabling and encouraging it, potentially taking the dieter from a calorie deficit to a calorie surplus for that week, making their diet plan essentially redundant. Do not consider the food you eat on cheat days as bad, just high calorific value. It can still be eaten if accounted for.

Why are they not needed for weight loss?

Many people who are trying to lose weight more than likely have an issue with overeating or binging already. Adding a 'cheat day' is just enabling them to carry on doing what got them into the situation they are now trying to escape from.

It is counterintuitive when you really break it down.

What is the alternative then?

As you know from chapter 2, calorie counting is the key to weight loss. Tracking calories in and calories out, to remain in a calorie deficit, is the most effective way to lose weight. So, what if you want that extra treat at the weekend? Let us say you are a female in a calorie deficit, consuming about 1800 calories a day (or 12,600 calories a week) and you fancy a pizza and a pint on Sunday which is 600 calories (bear in mind this is just an example because no pizza pint combo is that low in calories unfortunately). If you plan this into your diet schedule you can reduce your calorie intake for the first six days of the week by 100 calories a day leaving you at 12,000 by the end of the week. This extra 600-calorie deficit you have built up during the week can now account for your pizza and beer without taking you over your 12,600 calories a week target, leaving you in an overall calorie deficit. The added benefit of this is the lack of guilt. You have not broken your diet the way you would have with a conventional cheat day because it is part of your diet plan.

Chapter 5: Exercise

Increased physical activity helps burn more calories and raise your basal metabolic rate (BMR). Things as simple as taking stairs instead of the lift and parking further away from stores are small but powerful changes you can make on your weight loss journey. However, structured exercise programmes do far more for long-term fitness and weight loss.

A great exercise plan looks different for everyone. What you do depends on your weight, current health, age, abilities, and interests. No matter what physical condition you are currently in, you can start an exercise plan to lose excess fat, reduce the risk of serious health issues, and look and feel your best every day.

In chapter 6 we will talk about how a sedentary lifestyle contributes to unhealthy weight gain and a whole host of other physical and mental challenges. While boosting overall physical activity throughout the day makes quite a difference for your metabolism, a structured exercise programme does even better.

This does not mean you have to follow a celebrity fitness instructor's precise workout plan or spend hours pumping iron in the gym every day. All it means is to adopt a regular schedule of different exercise types that you enjoy, to help you achieve your weight loss and health goals.

Top Benefits of Structured Workouts on a Schedule

Not every advantage of a personalized fitness programme has to do with maximizing weight loss or improving your health and physique. Most are tangential to these overall goals. However, the type of structure that encourages long-term compliance with an exercise regimen also helps you lose weight and keep it off.

1 - Efficient Use of Time - Vague plans to increase physical activity throughout the day can leave you feeling rushed or unorganized. When you meet with a trainer or use your own research skills to create a structured exercise programme, you do not waste any time trying to figure out what to do and when to do it.

2 - A Healthy Mix of Targets - You do not need to be a bodybuilder to realize benefits from weight-training exercises. Aerobic exercises like brisk walking or bicycling do not only benefit endurance athletes. Create a structured exercise habit that incorporates all types of physical fitness to target different goals. For example, a jog or swimming laps improves cardiovascular health and burns more calories whilst building muscle mass promotes an increase in your metabolism, among other benefits.

3 - Set Schedules Beat the Need for Motivation - Too many people fail in their weight loss efforts because they do not set goals that make sense. Instead, they tried to use motivation or inspiration as the engine that drives their efforts. With structure and schedules, you create healthy habits from your to-do list just like any other chore or task.

4 - Structure and Goals Boosts Success - Taking a walk for 30 minutes every day at 4:00 PM is an example of a smart goal for a structured exercise plan. Going to the gym and completing a pre-planned routine is another. These goals are easier to track and succeed at than vague weight loss plans because they have concrete criteria. With the added side benefit that when you do tick them off your daily plan it will boost your motivation to continue hitting your targets.

What are the best exercises for weight loss?

This is a broad topic with many points and exercises I could cover but this book being a short guide, I will talk about my five favourite exercises for weight loss. It is important to remember that exercise alone will not help you lose weight. It needs to be balanced with a healthy, calorie deficit diet. No matter how much you exercise, if you are consuming more calories than you are burning you will not lose weight.

1. Walking. Walking is hands down one of the best exercises you can do for weight loss and for good reason too. It is easy, accessible, low impact (meaning less stress on your joints) and beginner friendly. There is no need to buy any equipment and the ability to start exercising without feeling overwhelmed, the way you might stepping onto the gym floor by yourself for the first time is priceless. Taking up more walking is a fantastic first step for anyone's weight loss journey. A 12-week study into the effects of walking on persons with obesity found that by walking three times a week for 50-70 minutes, waist circumference and body fat reduced by an average of 1.1 inches and 1.5% respectively[1].

2. Now my personal favourite form of exercise, weight training. Now you may not have expected weight training to be in this book for weight loss, but it is, and for good reason. Although a weight training session does not typically burn as many calories as a cardio workout of the same length may it is the other effects that are important. Weight training is more effective at building muscle than cardio is. An increase in muscle mass is linked to an increase in your resting metabolic rate (RMR) as muscle burns more calories than other tissues. To put this into perspective, a study was conducted to measure resting metabolism over a 24-week period of weight training. Weight training led to a 9% increase in resting metabolism for men and almost 4% for women. This increase is significant, but it is also important to understand how many calories this equates to. For men, it is about 140

additional calories burned a day whilst for women it is only 50 per day. This may not sound a lot, and it is not on its own however, with perspective and remembering that weight loss is not a one-day affair, rather a journey of potentially years and a complete lifestyle change. This daily increase can have a significant long-term impact on how quickly you reach your goals. Weight training has other significant calorie burning benefits. Specifically, that resting metabolism can remain elevated for up 38 hours after weight training, whilst no similar increase has been recorded for cardio[2].

3. HIIT or high intensity interval training is something I am all too familiar with being in the military. It is a PTIs favourite, and it is easy to see why. A typical HIIT workout lasts between 10-30 minutes and can burn a lot of calories and from one study, HIIT

burned 25-30% more calories per minute than weight training, running on a treadmill and cycling[3]. For me there are a few great benefits past their calorie burning effects. For one, they are easy to incorporate into your exercise routine, you pick an exercise, decide on your work and rest times then you are ready to start. For example, running as fast as you can for 30 seconds followed by walking at a steady pace for one to two minutes and repeat this pattern for 10-30 minutes. The second reason HIIT is a good choice for weight loss is the rest period. It allows for what I call a "you work, I work" routine. This is when you are exercising with someone else, which is a fantastic way to exercise as having someone else with you to push you and motivate you is always encouraging. One of you will perform your exercise of choice whilst the other rests for the same period. You then switch and so this pattern continues until you reach your target time.

4. Swimming is on my list not only because of how many calories it has the potential to burn but because of its low-impact nature. Swimming is a great option for those who may have joint pain or injuries as well as helping improve flexibility[4]. But do not be fooled by its low impact nature, per 30 minutes an average person can burn 372 calories doing breaststroke. So, it is still a fantastic form of exercise for weight loss[5].

5. Pilates is the final form of exercise on my list. If I were writing this a few years ago, it most likely would not have been included. I took up Pilates to try and help reduce my lower back pain and it has helped. However, that is not the only area of my

health that I saw improvement in. I saw significant improvements in my flexibility and balance. This in turn has helped improve my weight training performance in exercises such as squats where flexibility and range of motion are incredibly important. So, you may be thinking that Pilates is not for you since you do not do any weight training however Pilates itself does burn calories. An average person during a 30-minute Pilates class can burn 108 calories which is great considering it is beginner-friendly and for some more enjoyable than aerobic exercises making it easier to stick to especially since you can do it in the comfort of your own living room.

This is a short list for a short guide and as such has missed many forms of exercise.

I would encourage everyone to try and find a form of exercise they enjoy and make it a part of their weekly routine and stick to it. If it is fun, you will want to keep doing it. Consistency is the key for weight loss in general and in terms of exercise so if you find you are enjoying a form of exercise less and less then try something new, just do not give up.

How Often Should You Exercise for Weight Loss

Fitness and health experts may recommend a general number of hours or days per week that an adult should exercise for weight loss and overall health. However, the number would only be a generalised suggestion. As with most things, the exact answer depends on a variety of factors including your current weight, age, ability level, and how many calories you eat every day.

Most people agree that a battle against obesity is either won or lost in the kitchen. This means that what you eat and how many calories you consume matters a lot more than the amount of exercise you do. Another common saying is that you cannot out exercise a bad diet.

All that being said, a regular and structured exercise habit provides a long list of benefits that can help you lose weight and keep it off permanently. Remember that the goal is not to get to a certain number on the scale. It is to stay at a healthy weight for the rest of your life.

Determine Your Best Exercise Frequency

Losing weight always starts with figuring out how many calories you need to maintain your body. Then, you develop a diet and exercise plan that results in a calorie deficit, which means you consume fewer calories than you spend. How often you exercise and for how long affects how many calories you burn every day and over time. This is a good way to determine how often you should hit the gym, go out for a walk, or get involved with some other structured physical activity.

For adults without any serious health conditions managed by a doctor, the World Health Organization suggests a minimum of 2 ½ hours of exercise every week[6]. These 150 minutes, or approximately half an hour every workday, represent the minimum that will help you maintain reasonable fitness and reduce your chance of cardiovascular disease, diabetes, stroke, and other awful possibilities. Remember this is a suggested minimum and everybody should be aiming to exceed this whenever possible.

If you want to lose weight, the more exercise you do, the better. Half an hour every day will burn at least a couple of hundred calories depending on your weight and how rigorously you move. That can contribute to an extra pound of fat loss per week if you already eat at a deficit.

How often you exercise depends partly on how many calories you want to burn. However, you should not exercise for hours every day in an effort to lose weight more quickly. Instead, adjust your eating habits as more calories are burned from being active each day in comparison to those burned directly from exercise. When scheduling a new fitness habit, make it reasonable and suitable for your other life responsibilities. An hour at the gym is a way to take time for yourself, but if you keep adding more and more time, other aspects of your life may suffer. This is a balance that can take time to get right.

Chapter 6: Get Up and Move

With the increase in sit-down jobs, TV and computer entertainment, and more comfortable lifestyles, daily activity levels have fallen over the past few decades. Simple activities of daily living that used to fill our time and burn more calories have been replaced by more sedentary pastimes.

If you want to lose weight and improve overall health, increasing your daily activity levels makes sense. Just like you do not have to reach for a questionable weight loss pill or force yourself to follow a fad diet, you do not have to run a marathon or become a bodybuilder to lose unwanted pounds.

Regular exercise helps your body and mind in innumerable ways. However, if you are overweight or obese, have health problems, and have not exercised in a while, simply getting active is a great first step. It all has to do with the only true way to lose weight: calorie deficit. More activity equals more calories burned, and less excess stored as fat.

<u>Less Activity Equals More Unwanted Pounds</u>

It makes logical sense that sitting around and not exercising makes you burn fewer calories. If you do not restrict caloric intake enough, your body does not burn the extra fuel and instead transforms it into fat. This is all part of your natural metabolism. Various systems including the digestive tract and the hormone-producing endocrine system all play a role.

You cannot argue with basic maths. Too many calories that you do not burn equal excess weight. Besides storing body fat, an inactive or sedentary lifestyle has far-reaching effects on overall health and well-being.

<u>The Negative Impact of a Sedentary Lifestyle</u>

Sedentary means a tendency to spend most of your time seated or otherwise inactive. A sedentary lifestyle does not include regular physical activity or much if any structured exercise or fitness routines. If you work behind a computer, watch a lot of TV in the evenings, put your feet up to enjoy your hobby, or spend a lot of time driving or riding on public transport, you fit the criteria.

What negative health issues could you experience if you do not get enough daily physical activity[1].

- Physical Effects - As mentioned above, a sedentary lifestyle reduces the number of calories you burn every day and thus leads to weight gain. Also, you increase the risk of cardiovascular problems, insulin resistance, muscle and bone density loss, and a weakened immune system.

Using less energy leads to feeling worse, which feeds into a vicious cycle of becoming more sedentary over time. Anyone carrying extra weight knows that being active is more difficult. Compounding the physical effects of a sedentary lifestyle makes battling obesity harder.

- Mental and Emotional Effects - Multiple research studies also show that sitting around too much affects how you think and feel[2]. A sedentary way of life can contribute to depression, anxiety, increased stress levels, and overall lack of personal satisfaction and motivation. Being overweight in a world that focuses on physical attractiveness can already negatively influence your moods and emotional well-being. You do not need a lack of physical activity contributing to these problems.

Make Small Changes to Boost Weight Loss

Joining a gym, taking up a sport, or starting a regimented fitness routine are great ideas as long as your doctor clears you for that level of activity. However, you do not have to make drastic changes to your lifestyle to reap benefits. Simple changes that grow into daily habits will add up to a faster metabolism and a higher rate of burning calories.

A large part of overcoming a sedentary lifestyle involves changing your mindset to seek out opportunities to get active. If you want to change your weight and overall health, it helps to replace negative habits with more positive ones.

<u>Simple Changes for an Active Lifestyle</u>

Adopt one or more of these easy lifestyle changes to boost activity levels and read your calorie-burning engines. They will all help you lose weight, improve whole-body health, and decrease the risk of serious issues like stroke, diabetes, and depression.

1 - Walk More - Add an evening walk to your schedule, or simply increase opportunities to get up on your feet. Choose a parking spot further away from the shop or your workplace. Take your dog for an extra walk instead of just letting them run in the garden. If you do not have a dog and this is something you feel would motivate you, consider volunteering your time at a local animal shelter.

2 - Weight Bearing Exercise - While this may sound like a fitness regimen, it really focuses on you picking your own body weight up more often. Take the stairs instead of a lift. Stand up from your seat at least every hour. Carry luggage, gardening tools, or groceries in your hands instead of using a trolly. Consider using a standing desk instead of a traditional one with a chair. Even standing and shifting your weight can help burn more calories and combat circulatory problems.

3 - Pace and Fidget - While tapping your pencil or bouncing your knee will not make you lose weight on their own, the more general activity you work into your day, the better. Instead of lounging on the couch during a phone call, get up and pace across the room. Instead of lying down in bed to watch a movie, consider knitting, putting together a model, or engaging in some other minor activity at the same time.

4 - Make Time to Play - Video or computer games are fun, but they contribute to a sedentary lifestyle. Find new ways to play that get you up and moving. You do not have to be a fanatic to play a sport. Find a for-fun community 5-a-side league, take a tennis class or go bowling. Unstructured play works great, too. Throw a ball for your dog. Take a dip in the pool. Turn on some music and dance around your house like no one is watching. You will stay more active if you make it fun.

No matter what you decide to change, reinforce your new, more active lifestyle with reminders, goals, and schedules. Structured classes, teams, and events make this easy. You can use a simple calendar app to send notifications when you should stand up, take your dog for an extra walk, or engage in any of the other activities you want to try.

Chapter 7: Water

The human body is made up of about 60% water, so it stands to reason that it is the healthiest drink for you[1]. Water provides many benefits beyond quenching thirst. This non-calorific and non-nutritional beverage plays a vital role in weight loss efforts and ongoing weight management.

How much water should you drink every day? Does water really provide health benefits or is it just a replacement for higher calorie beverages? The facts may convince you to change your drinking habits completely.

The Role of Water in A Diet

Every part of your body needs water to function properly. While you get a portion of necessary hydration from the food you eat, drinking pure water is more effective. Dehydration can cause potentially serious health issues. Even a minor degree of dehydration can leave you feeling sluggish, tired, dizzy, and dull[2].

<u>Main Processes Helped by Proper Hydration</u>

Since the human body has such a high percentage of water in it, it makes sense that proper hydration affects everything. If you need additional inspiration to drink enough water every day, consider these physiological benefits.

1 - Removal of Waste Products - All cellular activity and metabolic activity creates waste. It is transported by your bloodstream, filtered by your kidneys and liver, and released from your body by respiration, perspiration, and through the digestive tract. Water makes the entire process work more smoothly, improves blood flow, facilitates kidney function, and helps to prevent urinary insufficiency and constipation.

2 - Protection for Spine and Joints - Water is your body's best lubricant for cells, tissues, and larger structures. It cushions and protects all moving parts. The synovial fluid that directly lubricates your joints is made up primarily of water. This fluid reduces the friction between joints and helps to maintain healthy tissue and joints.

3 - Promotes a Healthy Cardiovascular System - Your blood is mostly water, and you need sufficient hydration to help the red and white blood cells, platelets, electrolytes, and hormones flow through your body efficiently. Drinking enough water can help lower blood pressure, which contributes to a decreased risk of cardiovascular problems.

4 – Triggers Fullness and Aids in a Healthy Diet – When it comes to losing weight and optimizing your health, water plays an important role. Proper hydration can minimize feelings of hunger and influence how many calories you eat every day[3].

5 – Reduces Water Retention – It may seem counterintuitive to drink more water if you are retaining it in your body. If you properly hydrate, however, it signals your body to release stored water more effectively. This process is natural, healthy, and can help minimize bloating and the appearance of weight gain.

The numerous benefits of drinking enough water would create a very long list. When it comes to reducing calorie intake and losing weight, you cannot go wrong with this healthy beverage.

How Water Affects Food Consumption

Proper hydration with pure water affects how much food you eat in two different ways. It also offers a simple way to reduce the number of calories you have in your everyday diet. Many sources recommend eight glasses of water every day for a healthy adult. When it comes to people trying to lose fat and get to a healthy weight, water may be the "magical potion" that changes how much food and calorific beverages you consume every day.

- Water Has No Calories or Physiological Triggers - Consuming fewer calories than you burn is the only way to lose weight effectively. When you drink water, the ultimate zero calorie beverage, you naturally reduce the number of calories you consume. It is far too easy to drink excess calories if you reach for fruit juice, soda, beer or wine, or coffee and tea throughout the day.

Other no- or super low-calorie beverages exist. These include unsweetened tea, black coffee, and diet drinks flavoured with artificial sweetener. The first two have a negligible effect on your calorie intake or physiological reactions unless they contain caffeine. Drinks with artificial sweetener, however, may save you calories in the moment but could encourage increased intake later on[4].

You could fall into the trap of overcompensating for a perceived calorie deficit. If you order a diet soda with your meal, you may feel like you have freed up more calories from your daily target, allowing you to get a larger burger than you otherwise would have. Since you need a calorie deficit to lose weight, tricking your mind into eating more calories makes no sense. Stick with water and healthy portion sizes instead.

Second, artificial sweetener use can actually trigger the same reactions as eating or drinking real sugar. It seems that the sweet flavour itself starts your body's process of storing energy just like it would if it had a burst of glucose fuel instead[5]. This leads to a lower metabolic rate, more stored fat, and difficulty losing weight. Water and other unsweetened beverages do not create this physiological response.

Finally, excessively sweet foods train your taste buds to respond to sweetness more than other flavours. This reduces your ability to taste other foods accurately, which makes it harder to enjoy a healthy salad or chicken and vegetable stir fry. It gets harder to eat unsweetened foods because your sense of taste is not accustomed to unsweetened foods.

- Drinking Water Helps You Feel Full - Your body has an intricate system that lets you know when you are hungry or thirsty. A full stomach actually releases chemical signals that tell your brain to stop eating, I will go into more detail about this in chapter 9. For many overweight people, this system does not work as well as it should. You may lack a feeling of fullness even when you have eaten a reasonable meal.

If you drink two glasses of water 15 to 20 minutes before mealtime, you end up feeling fuller before you consume more calories than you need[6]. This not only affects your body chemistry and makes the natural process work more efficiently, but it helps you psychologically as well. If your stomach is full of water, you cannot eat as much food. A satisfied and full feeling reduces your desire to snack or reach for high-calorie foods and beverages.

- Proper Hydration Helps You Stay on Track Mentally - Since dehydration can affect your mood and cognitive ability, it makes sense that drinking enough water keeps you sharp and focused. Lowered impulse control makes it far too easy to reach for a sugary snack or choose unhealthy options when presented with a choice between take-away pizza and a delicious salad.

Water makes it easier for you to stick to your weight loss plan and stay motivated every day. It may even reduce the stress hormone cortisol response, which also triggers overeating[7]. This is especially true for people who exercise regularly or have recently increased physical activity.

<u>The Link Between Water and Physical Performance/Everyday Activity</u>

You know how important staying active is for your weight loss journey. Exercise or simple active lifestyle changes burn more calories, rev up your metabolism, and provide a host of other health benefits. Water makes positive changes in this aspect of your new, healthy lifestyle, too.

- Hydration Supports Muscle and Joint Movement and Health - Increase physical performance and reduce the risk of soreness or injury by drinking plenty of water every day. Dehydration happens more easily through respiration and perspiration when you are working out. Always take a bottle of fresh water to the gym or on a walk around the neighbourhood. Drinking water keeps your muscle tissues, joints, tendons and ligaments, and other moving parts well-lubricated. It can also reduce the risk of cramps.

- Water Improves Cardiovascular Performance
- Your lungs, heart, and entire circulatory system works harder when you exercise. Without sufficient water in your system, these organs will not work as efficiently. This can raise blood pressure to unhealthy levels, increase your heart rate and cause undue strain on your entire body's systems.

Without enough water intake, your overall physical capabilities decrease[8]. You will not be able to do enough exercise to make a difference in your calorie use. This does not mean that the more water you drink, the more exercise you can do. You need to drink enough to keep your body in proper working condition. This will make increased physical activity easier, healthier, and more comfortable.

The Link Between Water and Weight Loss

The list of reasons why drinking water helps weight loss can stretch on for miles. This non-calorific beverage affects all systems in your body, from the actions you perform to the choices you make. The link between water and weight loss is as strong as the link between hydrogen and oxygen molecules that make up this precious liquid. Water is simple, accessible, affordable, portable, and can help you look and feel your very best.

The #1 Lifestyle Change You Can Make

When you drink water as part of your weight loss efforts, you change so many things about how your body feels and functions. Choosing a non-calorific beverage that does not trigger a metabolic response reduces overall calorie consumption and keeps your body running smoothly. It does not add extra calories to your diet, so you will not store any more as fat. In the simple calories in, calories out equation, cutting back on the first part is the easiest.

Water keeps all your systems running properly and maintains proper metabolic function. Even if you do not change the number of calories you consume, drinking water helps your body use them more efficiently. You also flush out waste products and regulate your digestive system at the same time.

Do not underestimate water when it comes to keeping you on track with your new habits. Dehydration leads to cognitive functional difficulties that may actually increase the chance of snacking or choosing sugary or starchy foods. Although a couple of glasses of water will not automatically switch your tastes to grilled vegetables and chicken breast, it contributes to your overall mental well-being.

When you feel your best and your body operates optimally, making lifestyle changes that stick is so much easier. Your weight loss journey may take many months or even years. If you want to maintain a healthy weight for your entire life, you cannot return to excessive calorie consumption and a sedentary lifestyle. You also cannot go back to drinking high-calorie sodas, sugary fruit juices, or alcoholic beverages like beer and wine to excess.

If any secret formula or magic trick exists in the world of weight loss, it is water. Forget trendy energy drinks or diet beverages with artificial sweeteners. Even if they cut calories, they do not contribute to overall health. Water is simply the best option for losing weight and keeping it off forever.

Chapter 8: Mindset and Motivation

Websites, social media groups, in-person meetings, health programmes, and weight loss organizations all exist to provide support and motivation to people who struggle with unwanted pounds. The motivation and accountability parts of the entire diet and fitness industries represent a considerable portion of those £2 billion I mentioned at the start of this book. While outside support can help you stay on track, it is essential that you adopt the right mindset for long-term success.

Too many diets and fitness programs focus on the next 30 days or maybe a few months. Expectations of pounds down and meeting target weights keep you motivated for a short period of time. However, when you find that you have not achieved all your goals at the end of the limited timeframe, you may feel let down. When the programme ends, you may return to your old way of eating and a lower daily activity level only to find that the pounds start rolling back on.

Mindset matters when it comes to achieving your desired healthy weight. If you want to make lifelong changes to look and feel your best every day, calorie-controlled eating and increased activity must become a permanent lifestyle change.

<u>Find Your "Why"</u>

Calorie counting and deficit leads to weight loss. This scientific fact holds true for everyone who struggles with excess pounds. The process is simple but losing weight and keeping it off is still not necessarily easy. If it were, the world would not be struggling with a growing obesity epidemic.

Your personal journey to a healthy and vigorous self starts with the knowledge shared in this book. You now understand why counting calories works and how to do it effectively, as well as other aspects to leading a healthy lifestyle. However, knowing how and putting the practice into effect are two very different things. Many experts speak about finding your why or your reason to lose weight. This personal understanding can fuel your efforts in the beginning.

<u>What "Whys" Exist for Weight Loss</u>

Although everyone has their own story and personal reasons for changing their life, most list one of these three when it comes to losing weight.

1 - Health and Longevity - Excess weight is not healthy. While the majority understands this, people may struggle with making a change until something drastic happens. Your doctor may diagnose you with prediabetes or high blood pressure. You may experience health complications with an existing illness. Perhaps you just hate the way you get out of breath when climbing stairs or playing with your kids. One of the top reasons to lose weight involves improving health and making sure you stay healthy and active for many years to come.

2 - Improved Appearance - There is nothing vain or shallow about wanting to look your best. You may feel more attractive and happier without the extra pounds.

3 - Confidence and Value - Good health and attractiveness help boost confidence and your sense of self-worth. That does not mean that overweight people have less value than slender ones. Even though society may perceive this as truth, it is an uncomfortable and unfair assumption. That being said, achieving weight loss goals and transforming your life will surely boost your confidence. You may want to do this to help others in the future or become a positive role model for family and friends.

Do you need a big reason to lose weight? No. If you cut calories and increase your activity level, you can lose weight without some grand motivating factor. You will receive the benefits anyway.

Is having a strong why enough for a lifelong change? Probably not.

Why a Reason Is Not Always Enough

Even the best reasons to start a weight loss journey may not carry you through to success and healthy maintenance for the rest of your life. Just like a spark can start a fire, you need to constantly fuel it if you want to stay warm. Mental or emotional fuel for a lifelong fight against obesity cannot come from one idea at the start.

People struggle with their weight, get caught in a cycle of yo-yo dieting, and often regain everything even if they lost it in a healthy manner before.

Some studies have indicated that an average of 80% of people who lose weight are likely to gain it back[1].

How do you avoid becoming part of this unfortunate statistic? Do not expect your initial reason to keep your mind on task every time you are faced with a doughnut or an opportunity to laze around on the couch. Lifelong changes require lifelong habits.

Make Healthy Changes a Lifelong Plan

This is where most fad diets, "quick weight loss tricks," and secret celebrity fat busting plans fall apart. Besides the fact that they are all just cleverly marketed calorie counting, most promise results in a specific period of time. Follow this food plan for 30 days to a brand-new you. See the difference a week can make. Just six weeks will erase years of bad eating. These kinds of claims offer unrealistic expectations.

You do not want to lose weight for 30 days or six weeks. You want to lose weight and keep it off for the rest of your life. Yes, some special programme may help you lose weight for a period of time. The instant the plan ends, you go right back to your old habits and regain everything.

Permanent Changes Require Lifelong Habits

Creating these habits requires more than initial enthusiasm, a strong why, and big dreams. To improve your health, get rid of unwanted fat, avoid weight-related health problems, and feel your best forever, long-term habits mean so much more than even the strongest spark of motivation.

These five tips will help you create lifelong change:

1 - Acceptance - Before you do anything else, you need to accept that you have to change your eating and activity habits forever. Get over the idea that you will lose weight quickly and it will stay off even if you go back to your old lifestyle.

2 - Make Actionable Goals - Instead of focusing on a specific number on the scale or a time limit, create goals based on actions, and new habits. For example, make it your goal to track the calories for everything you eat every day. Another great goal would be to take a walk three times every week. Make it achievable, specific and most importantly be consistent in achieving it.

3 - Track and Record - Count calories, keep track of activity, and consider writing in a journal to record your moods, motivation, and struggles. Do not let higher calories or your former sedentary lifestyle creep up on you without noticing. The more you keep track, the easier it is to stay on track.

4 - Practice Patience - Weight loss and improved health is not a race. While everyone wants to look and feel their best as soon as possible, you cannot create sustainable habits with a time limit in mind. If your goal is to track calories to maintain a healthy weight for the rest of your life, no end date exists when you can stop.

5 - Celebrate Success - When you succeed with your actionable goals, celebrate with a non-food reward. Maintaining a positive attitude about your weight loss journey is an important part of exceeding for the long term. Get a massage or a new tattoo. Buy yourself a piece of jewellery or a new tool for your garage. This positive reinforcement of your achievements will provide a significant boost to your motivation. Take time to recognize your efforts in counting calories, tracking food, or increasing activity levels. These are the things that will allow you to live a long life at a healthy weight.

Chapter 9: Sleep

How much sleep is required each night?

The phrase 'a good night's sleep' has long been used as a recommendation for optimum health and wellbeing, but what it truly means is not 100% clear. Sleep is not a cure-all for illness or disorder, of course, but it affects how your entire body functions and operates. It is also important for weight loss and maintaining a healthy weight once you achieve it.

Learn how to define what a good night's sleep is for you, its connection to losing weight, and how to achieve one every night.

How much sleep you need varies depending on age but for a healthy adult, it is recommended to have between six and eight hours of sleep a night. I often work night shifts so, me telling you to have a regular sleep pattern and to get a certain amount of sleep each night may seem hypocritical but, it is because I work the unsociable hours, that I fully understand how important and valuable sleep is for weight loss, physical performance, and mental health.

According to a study published by the International Journal of Obesity, those who slept between six and eight hours had a better chance of losing weight and achieving their target than those who had less than six hours of sleep a night.

The study was a six-month intensive weight loss intervention programme for 472 obese adults. This study found that participants who slept between six and seven or seven and eight hours a night were more likely to lose at least 4.5kg than those who slept for six hours or less a night[1].

Quality of Sleep

The length of time you stay asleep is not the only important factor in your overall health. Quality of sleep also matters. In the discussion about fighting obesity and maintaining a healthy body weight, average sleep numbers and good sleep habits are excellent targets you can set yourself. What this specifically means for you needs closer consideration.

<u>Create a Specific Sleep Number for You</u>

First, consider your age. If you are over 18, you should aim to get at least seven hours of sleep every night. However, you may feel better with eight or even nine hours. Part of determining how much sleep you need comes down to trial and error. If you do not feel refreshed after seven hours, add another hour to your nightly rest.

Other signs you need more sleep include:

- Over-reliance on caffeine or energy drinks.
- Increased appetite.
- Moodiness and irritability.
- Reduced cognitive function, memory, and focus.
- Dark circles under your eyes or a dull complexion.

Multiple studies have suggested that the amount of time spent in the different stages of sleep is equally important as the total amount of time spent asleep.

 A study in 2009 found that those who got less slow-wave sleep had an increased risk of obesity, even when controlling the total sleep time[2].

So, how can you improve your quality of sleep?

Well, here are some of my tips to help improve your quality of sleep during your weight loss journey:

- **Set that alarm early:** Those with a late bedtime may consume more calories and be at a higher risk of weight gain[3]. So, going to sleep and waking up earlier than you normally would, may be beneficial for your weight loss.

- **Sleep in a dark room:** This may sound like I am teaching you to suck eggs, but it is something I am guilty of and I know many others are too. I find myself staring at my phone just before I go to sleep and this artificial light exposure, whether it be from a phone, tv, or lamp, can slow or even halt the production of melatonin. Melatonin being the natural hormone that promotes sleep and helps regulate our circadian rhythm (circadian rhythm is the natural and internal process that regulates your body's sleep-wake cycle). Therefore, avoiding bright lights close to your bedtime can improve the length and quality of your sleep.

- **Do not consume food close to bedtime:** Studies have shown that consuming food later in the day and close to bedtime can reduce the success rate of weight loss[4].

- **Maintain a regular sleep schedule:** An inconsistent sleep schedule or using the weekend to catch up on sleep that you missed during the week can negatively impact your metabolism and reduce insulin sensitivity, allowing blood sugar levels to become elevated. I will expand on this point in more detail later in this chapter.

- **Reduce stress:** We have all had nights where it feels like your mind just will not switch off and falling asleep can become frustrating. It is during times like these that I like to use mindfulness to help alleviate this by reducing stress and anxiety, ultimately helping me fall asleep.

<u>The importance of a consistent sleep schedule</u>

A regular and consistent sleep schedule is more significant for weight loss than you may initially believe. An irregular or poor sleep schedule can promote metabolic dysregulation as well as insulin resistance through prolonged elevated blood sugar, known as hyperglycaemia[5].

Why is insulin so important? Insulin is a hormone produced by the pancreas that transfers sugar from your blood into cells, where it can then be used for energy. Energy storage also involves insulin as it tells your cells when to store energy as fat or glycogen, the storage form of glucose.

Insulin resistance, which can develop from a poor sleep schedule, is when your cells no longer respond to insulin as they should. This leads to elevated sugar and insulin levels. Though cells become resistant to insulin's effect, they will still respond to the hormone's other role in storing fat and as a result fat storage is increased. Therefore, insulin resistance combined with high blood sugar levels are connected to increased body fat levels.

<u>Connection between weight and sleep</u>

A lot of information exists that pairs weight loss efforts to sleep habits. These often focus on snacking more if you stay up late, not eating too close to bedtime to boost your metabolism and consuming less sugar, and high-calorie caffeinated beverages to get you through the day.

Lack of sleep has a more direct correlation to actions and decisions that promote weight gain from a physiological standpoint, however[6].

- Poor Sleep Decreases Impulse Control - If your body and mind do not get enough rest, your cognitive ability suffers. The frontal lobe, which is responsible for conscious decision making, gets sluggish and does not work as well. Therefore, you are physiologically incapable of resisting temptation or making a smart choice between a salad and a slice of pizza.

- Lack of Sleep Reduces the Serotonin Response - The natural feel-good chemicals in your brain give you a continuous reward throughout the day and a boost when something pleasurable happens. This could include laughing at a great joke, kissing a loved one, or eating a delicious piece of chocolate. When you do not get enough sleep, your serotonin response is interrupted. This forces your brain to look for more rewards to maintain a higher sense of pleasure. Yummy snacks are quite easy to reach for and do the job well. People report increased cravings for carb-rich, high-calorie foods when they are sleep deprived.

- The Cortisol Response Triggers - Cortisol is a stress hormone that is closely tied to unhealthy weight gain and other physical issues. When you experience a spike in cortisol, your body goes into a type of survival mode and begins storing as many calories as possible. If you do not get enough sleep, cortisol levels increase, and fat stores begin to build.

- Sleep Affects Insulin Production - If all that was not enough to convince you to get a good night's sleep, staying up too late or waking up too early also reduces insulin sensitivity. This means your body cannot process starch, sugars, and other nutrients as effectively as before. Your entire metabolism slows down, and even your normal number of calories can result in excess fat storage.

Not getting enough hours of sleep every day causes these changes in your body. However, studies show that high sleep variability also leads to negative consequences[7]. This term describes people who sleep at different times and for different lengths on different days. Your body works better if you get six to eight hours of sleep regularly every night than it does if you get six hours one night, nine hours the next, just four at the weekend, and 10 to "make up for it" the following day.

Impact of Sleep on Calorie Intake

The amount and quality of sleep has decreased over the years at the same time the rate of obesity has increased. This correlation may not prove causation at face value, but researchers have found more specific proof that sleep affects calorie intake and therefore weight gain.

When you do not sleep enough, you frequently adopt simple lifestyle changes like snacking more in the evening or grabbing a mocha latte or piece of chocolate to keep you going through the long afternoon. However, there are very real physical and chemical changes that occur in your body that practically force you to eat more calories.

As mentioned earlier, poor sleep habits decrease your ability to resist temptation, affect your natural serotonin and cortisol hormone levels, and change the insulin response. All of these things can encourage increased caloric intake.

Sleep and Hormones

Ghrelin and Leptin.

"What are these?", I hear you ask. Ghrelin and Leptin are hormones that are connected to appetite. The hormone Ghrelin promotes hunger and Leptin contributes to feeling full when eating. The body will naturally increase and decrease the levels of these hormones during the day, producing that feeling of hunger and the need to consume calories.

With the average self-reported sleep duration decreasing by 2 hours over the past 40 years, a study was conducted to establish the connection between sleep and weight in relation to Ghrelin and Leptin levels. The study concluded that with a decrease in sleep duration there is an associated increase in Ghrelin levels and a reduction in the levels of Leptin resulting in increased hunger and appetite[8].

Sleep and Calorie Intake

Ghrelin and Leptin may be an established connecting factor between weight and sleep, but they are not the only influence on weight.

A common factor of increased calorie intake is our inability to identify the signals our bodies are giving us. Many will often confuse boredom, tiredness, and even thirst for hunger.

This begins a cycle, when you eat something because you believe you are hungry but in fact, are just thirsty and then repeat this. Every time you are slightly thirsty it will prompt you to consume calories. It is this confusion of signals from our bodies that can be a contributing factor to weight gain, demonstrating the need for a carefully structured daily meal plan including drinking water, to help prevent yourself from misinterpreting your body's signals and consuming excess calories.

Sleep and Physical Activity Levels

You do not need a scientific research study to tell you that lack of sleep leaves you feeling tired and sluggish. You would rather nap or lounge around doing a simple activity rather than going to the gym, taking a walk, or engaging in other physical activities.

<u>Rest and Exercise Benefit Each Other</u>

If you get enough sleep, you have more energy to maintain a higher activity level. If you exercise, you also get better sleep. Physical activity and a healthy sleep habit go hand in hand[9]. Even if you do not feel energetic, taking a walk, lifting some weights, or dancing to your favourite song can interrupt the poor sleep/low energy cycle. In time, the enforced activity will improve how you feel all the time. Of course, it also helps boost your metabolism and contributes to healthy weight loss.

This does not mean you should adopt a strenuous fitness regime right before you go to bed every night. In fact, as with most exercise recommendations, ease into things to decrease the chance of injury or burnout. The amount of activity you need to improve your sleep habits depends largely on your current fitness levels and your age.

Moderate exercise often works better than more intense options. Simple stretching and low-weight resistance training can even help people with insomnia[10]. A 10-to-15-minute walk early in the day can set you up for a more restful night. Experts generally recommend no intense physical activity two to three hours before your expected bedtime. Good sleep habits happen when you stick to a regular schedule.

<u>Make a Change</u>

Whether you are reading this book for information on losing weight or ways to lead a healthier life, my advice is the same. Doing something is always better than doing nothing. Make a change in your life for the better and be consistent with it. No matter how small it may seem it will produce a big result.

If you make a consistent effort, no matter how small, you will achieve more than those who do nothing.

The effects of small changes and habits compound over time.

1% better each day for a year.

$$1.01^{365} = 37.78$$

1% worse every day for a year.

$$0.99^{365} = 00.03$$

You will end up with results that are 37 times better after one year if you can get just 1% better each day.

Life

Begins

At

The

End

Of

Your

Comfort

Zone.

-Neale Donald Walsch-

We all have that moment of fear and self-doubt when trying something new. I have always remembered this quote and it helps motivate and encourage me to push my boundaries at times like that. I hope these words will stick with you the way they have for me, next time you are in a new and unfamiliar situation.

So, when you close this book do not carry on with your days as normal. Make a change in your life, no matter how small it may seem.

References:

Chapter 1: Introduction

1 - https://www.prnewswire.com/news-releases/united-states-weight-loss-market-to-decline-by-9-to-71-billion-in-2020---assessment-of-the-changing-consumer-dieting-behavior-due-to-covid-19-301070748.html

2 - https://www.cdc.gov/obesity/data/adult.html

Chapter 2: Calorie counting

1 - https://www.livescience.com/52802-what-is-a-calorie.html

2 - https://pubmed.ncbi.nlm.nih.gov/24636238/

3 - https://www.healthline.com/nutrition/calories-in-calories-out#what-it-is

4 - http://news.bbc.co.uk/1/hi/health/4311087.stm#:~:text=Lacors%2C%20the%20body%20that%20advises,and%205%25%20of%20a%20food

Chapter 3: Portion Sizes

1 - https://www.ncbi.nlm.nih.gov/pmc/articles/PMC1447051/

2 - https://abcnews.go.com/WN/food-portion-sizes-grown-lot/story?id=129685#:~:text=%22The%20sizes%20of%20the%20increase,crackers%2C%20are%2060%20percent%20larger

3 - https://pescience.com/blogs/blog/portion-size

4 - https://my.clevelandclinic.org/health/articles/9436-controlling-portion-sizes

Chapter 5: Exercise

1 - https://pubmed.ncbi.nlm.nih.gov/25566464/

2 - https://link.springer.com/article/10.1007/s00421-001-0568-y?LI=true

3 - https://pubmed.ncbi.nlm.nih.gov/25162652/

4 - https://pubmed.ncbi.nlm.nih.gov/26535217/

5 - https://www.health.harvard.edu/diet-and-weight-loss/calories-burned-in-30-minutes-of-leisure-and-routine-activities

6- https://www.who.int/dietphysicalactivity/physical-activity-recommendations-18-64years.pdf

Chapter 6: Get up and move

1 - https://medlineplus.gov/healthrisksofaninactivelifestyle.html

2 - https://www.psychologytoday.com/us/blog/minding-the-body/201403/what-sitting-does-your-psyche

Chapter 7: water

1 - https://www.usgs.gov/special-topic/water-science-school/science/water-you-water-and-human-body?qt-science_center_objects=0#qt-science_center_objects

2 – https://www.nhs.uk/conditions/dehydration/

3 – https://onlinelibrary.wiley.com/doi/abs/10.1111/jhn.12368

4 – https://www.health.harvard.edu/blog/artificial-sweeteners-sugar-free-but-at-what-cost-201207165030

5 – https://www.medpagetoday.com/meetingcoverage/endo/71882

6 – https://www.ncbi.nlm.nih.gov/pmc/articles/PMC6209729/

7 – https://pubmed.ncbi.nlm.nih.gov/17006802/

8 - https://www.nature.com/articles/1601897

Chapter 8: Mindset and Motivation

1 - https://www.webmd.com/diet/news/20161014/how-your-appetite-can-sabotage-weight-loss#1

Chapter 9: Sleep

1 - https://pubmed.ncbi.nlm.nih.gov/21448129/

2 - https://academic.oup.com/sleep/article/32/4/483/2454374

3 - https://pubmed.ncbi.nlm.nih.gov/23814334/

4 - https://www.sleepfoundation.org/physical-health/weight-loss-and-sleep#:~:text=Sleep%20During%20Weight%20Loss,17%20and%20enco urage%20overeating18.

5 - https://pubmed.ncbi.nlm.nih.gov/30827911/

6 - https://www.ncbi.nlm.nih.gov/pmc/articles/PMC2951287/

7 - https://www.medicalnewstoday.com/articles/325629#Good-sleep-is-part-of-successful-weight-loss

8 - https://pubmed.ncbi.nlm.nih.gov/15583226/

9 - https://www.ncbi.nlm.nih.gov/pmc/articles/PMC4341978/

10 - https://www.scielo.br/scielo.php?script=sci_arttext&pid=S1516-44462019000100051&lng=en&nrm=iso&tlng=en

The information provided in this book is designed to provide helpful information on the subjects discussed. This book is not meant to be used, nor should it be used, to diagnose or treat any medical condition. For diagnosis or treatment of any medical problem, consult your own physician. The publisher and author are not responsible for any specific health or allergy needs that may require medical supervision and are not liable for any damages or negative consequences from any treatment, action, application or preparation to any person reading or following the information in this book. References are provided for informational purposes only and do not constitute an endorsement of any websites or other sources. Readers should be aware that the websites listed in this book may change.